CW00507315

Pocket Picture Guides

Head Injuries

Head Injuries

Peter J. Teddy DPhil FRCS
Consultant Neurosurgeon
Department of Neurological Surgery

Philip Anslow MA MB MChir FRCR
Senior Registrar in Neuroradiology

The Radcliffe Infirmary
Woodstock Road
Oxford, UK

J.B. Lippincott Company • Philadelphia
Gower Medical Publishing • London • New York

Distributed in USA and Canada by:

J. B. Lippincott Company
East Washington Square
Philadelphia, PA 19105
USA

Distributed in UK and Continental Europe by:

Harper & Row Ltd
Middlesex House
34-42 Cleveland Street
London W1P 5EB
UK

Distributed in Philippines/Guam, Middle East,
Latin America and Africa by:

Harper & Row International
East Washington Square
Philadelphia, PA 19105
USA

Distributed in Southeast Asia, Hong Kong,
India and Pakistan by:

Harper & Row Publishers (Asia) Pte Ltd
37 Jalan Pemimpin 02-01
Singapore 2057

Distributed in Japan by:

Igaku Shoin Ltd
Tokyo International
P.O. Box 5063
Tokyo
Japan

Distributed in Australia and New Zealand by:

Harper & Row (Australasia) Pty Ltd
P.O. Box 226
Artarmon, N.S.W. 2064
Australia

Library of Congress Catalog Number: 87-82129

British Library Cataloguing in Publication Data

Teddy, Peter J.
  Head Injuries.
  1. Man. Head. Injuries
  I. Title   II. Anslow, Philip   III. Series
  617′.51044

ISBN: 0-397-44569-5 (Lippincott/Gower)

Project Editor: Michele Campbell
Design: Marie McNestry

Produced by Mandarin Offset/
Printed in Hong Kong in 1989
Set in Sabon and Frutiger by Dawkins Typesetters, London.

CONTENTS

ACKNOWLEDGEMENTS

The authors wish to thank all their many colleagues who helped towards the production of this book by generously donating slides or radiographs from their personal or departmental collections. Particular thanks are due to Mr Michael Briggs, Consultant Neurosurgeon, Dr M Esiri and Dr M V Squier, Consultant Neuropathologists at the Radcliffe Infirmary, and to Dr Trudi Blamires, Registrar in Ophthalmology, and Mr Steven Vernon at the Oxford Eye Hospital for their generous assistance. We also wish to thank the patients who so kindly consented to their pictures being used for publication and Miss Sandra Cowdrey for her help in typing the manuscript.

INTRODUCTION

Many victims of severe injuries to the head who have the potential to make an excellent recovery from the primary brain injury may deteriorate or die for lack of prompt or adequate medical care of secondary insults to the brain, such as raised intracranial pressure, hypoxia and hypercarbia, hypotension, infection and epileptic fits. The indirect effects of injury to other parts of the body may also be overlooked in the presence of an apparently massive head injury. An important aspect in the treatment of head injuries is the identification of this group of patients, with anticipation of the potential complications and their prompt and proper correction.

Hospital management falls into several broad phases:
- emergency treatment and assessment of the (unconscious) patient;
- history-taking and examination;
- preliminary investigations and their interpretations;
- emergency medical and surgical treatment;
- transfer to neurosurgical units;
- further investigations;
- short-term management and rehabilitation.

This book is not a comprehensive text of the management of head injuries, but intends rather to reinforce pictorially the important underlying principles involved at each stage in the treatment of the more severe head injuries.

PATHOLOGICAL CONSIDERATIONS

The skull

Severe blows to the head deform the skull which, when the limits of its elasticity are exceeded, will fracture. Fractures may be linear, stellate or depressed, depending on the velocity of the blow and the size and contours of the applied surface. The fracture lines usually run from the centre of impact towards the base of the skull but also depend upon the contours and buttresses of the skull itself. Approximately eighty percent of fatally head-injured patients have skull fractures.

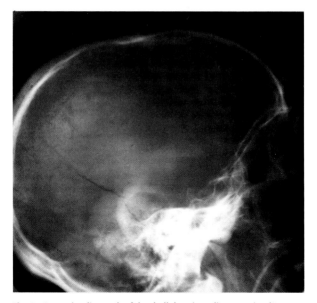

Fig. 1 Lateral radiograph of the skull showing a linear parietal/temporal fracture extending towards the base of the skull.

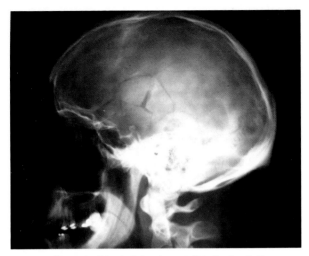

Fig. 2 Radiograph of the skull showing a stellate fracture in the temporoparietal region, the result of a blow from the legendary 'blunt instrument'.

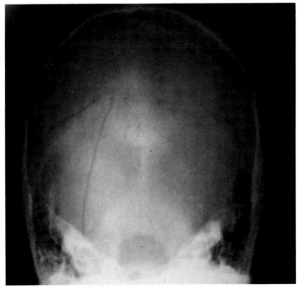

Fig. 3 Towne's view of the skull showing a right occipital fracture.

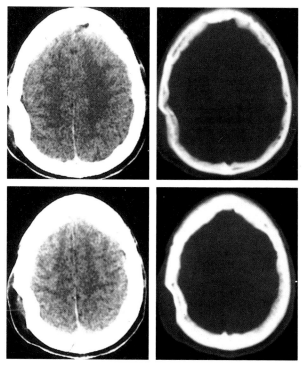

Fig. 4 Computerized tomographic (CT) scan of the skull showing a left posterior parietal depressed fracture with no suggestion of cortical damage beneath the fracture site.

Primary brain injury

The grey matter of the brain may be contused directly below the site of impact by inward deformation of the skull (a coup injury) or at distant sites through inertial pressure (contre-coup). The distribution of the latter injuries is related to the rigidity and irregularity of the inner surface of the skull, and to the dural partitions. The most frequent sites of such superficial injury, therefore, are the frontal and temporal poles, the undersurfaces of the temporal and frontal lobes, and those structures adjacent to the falx cerebri and tentorium cerebelli.

More diffuse injury to the brain is due to shear strain within cerebral tissue after impact, greatly exacerbated by rotation. Since the head is rarely in a fixed position at the time of injury, rotational acceleration/deceleration almost always occurs to some degree. The injury probably progresses centrally (from cortex to diencephalon to mesencephalon) depending on the severity of impact. In rapidly fatal injuries, the brain stem may be extensively damaged due to massive fracturing of the base of the skull. In cases of 'brain stem' injury with coma, decerebrate rigidity and autonomic disturbance, there is invariably not only disruption of the brain stem, but also much more widespread damage to the white matter.

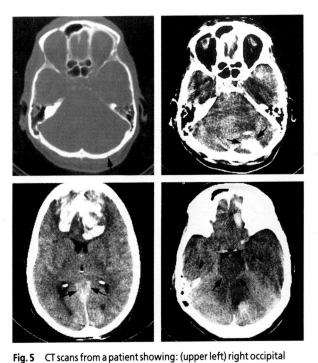

Fig. 5 CT scans from a patient showing: (upper left) right occipital fracture (arrow) with overlying boggy swelling; (upper right) right cerebellar contusion (arrow) in relation to the fracture (coup injury); (lower left & right) severe contrecoup injury to the frontal lobe and cerebral swelling (arrow) obliterating the cerebrospinal fluid (CSF) cisterns around the brain stem.

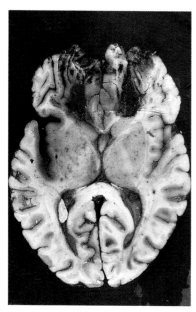

Fig. 6 Horizontal section showing severe frontal contusion and intracerebral haemorrhage following occipital injury similar to that in Figs 4 and 5, upper left.

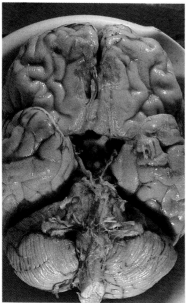

Fig. 7 Basal view showing typical damage to the frontal and temporal poles sustained in an acceleration/deceleration injury.

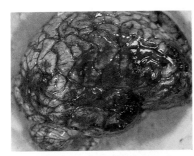

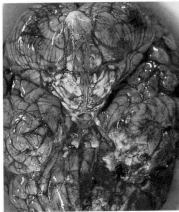

Fig. 8 Lateral (upper) and basal (lower) views showing subarachnoid haemorrhage and extensive damage to the undersurface of the brain, notably in the right temporal and subfrontal regions. These are typical contrecoup injuries from a blow to the left side of the head.

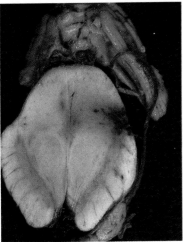

Fig. 9 Transverse section of brain stem showing extensive direct injury with haemorrhage and contusion.

Secondary injury to the brain

Subsequent to the primary brain injury, one or more of an often interrelated group of events may be superimposed and lead to deterioration in cerebral function through interference with the energy supply to the brain or through infection. Such factors include:

Raised intracranial pressure

The skull is effectively a closed box; thus, as the intracranial volume increases, so will pressure increase and tend to decrease cerebral perfusion. The main causes of increased intracranial pressure in head injuries are cerebral swelling and intracranial haemorrhage. Cerebral swelling ('oedema') is most frequently due to fluid passing into the extracellular spaces through damaged vascular endothelium.

Intracranial haemorrhage may occur within the extradural, subdural or subarachnoid spaces, or within the brain or ventricular system. Subarachnoid and intraventricular haemorrhage may in turn lead to impaired circulation and resorption of cerebrospinal fluid (CSF), thereby producing hydrocephalus with a secondary rise in intracranial pressure.

Ischaemic brain damage

This may be due to focal contusion with infarction, more generalized infarction (such as caused by occlusion of the posterior cerebral artery during transtentorial herniation) or even more diffuse infarction, as in fat embolism or following widespread injury.

Cerebral hypoxia and hypercarbia

These may be related to impaired gas exchange in the lungs or to impaired ventilation and may be important adverse factors in patients with chest infection, pulmonary oedema, shock lung, pneumohaemothorax, flail chest or multiple rib fractures, and in patients with prolonged epileptic fits. The effects of hypoxia and/or hypercarbia may be exacerbated by systemic hypotension with impaired cerebral blood flow.

Disordered cerebral autoregulation

The normal brain maintains its blood supply within fairly narrow limits, probably through myogenic autoregulation within cerebral vessels. The damaged brain loses this capacity to regulate its blood supply, and cerebral blood flow becomes more passively related to changes in systemic blood pressure. As cerebral perfusion pressure equals systemic arterial pressure minus intracranial pressure, any increase in intracranial pressure or drop in systemic pressure diminishes cerebral perfusion.

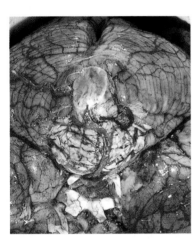

Fig. 10 Basal view showing severe uncal and cerebellar herniation secondary to acute bilateral subdural haematomas and generalized brain injury.

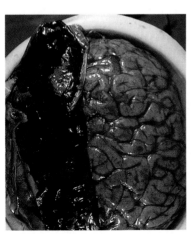

Fig. 11 Superior view showing extensive acute subdural haematoma over the right cerebral hemisphere.

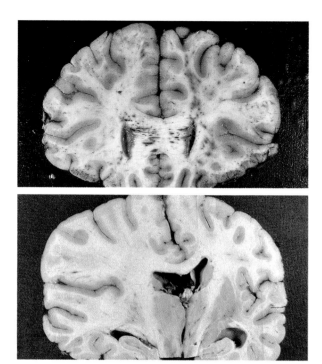

Fig. 12 Coronal sections from cases of severe closed primary head injuries showing (upper) widespread haemorrhage within the white matter and (lower) extensive cortical damage with extensive oedema of the right cerebral hemisphere and a midline shift to the left.

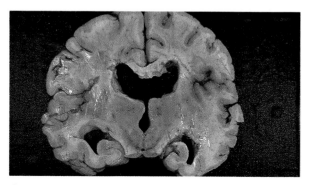

Fig. 13 Coronal section showing substantial ventricular dilatation due to severe hydrocephalus secondary to a primary head injury.

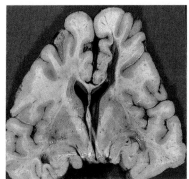

Fig. 14 Coronal section showing bilateral hemispheric compression due to bilateral subdural haematomas. Note the bilateral uncal herniation.

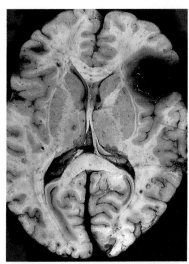

Fig. 15 Horizontal (upper) and coronal (lower) sections showing severe focal right frontal lobe injury caused by a low-velocity penetrating missile.

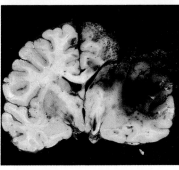

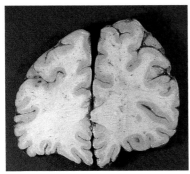

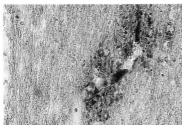

Fig. 16 Fat embolism: (upper) coronal section shows cerebral bleeding and scattered petechial haemorrhages in the cortex; (lower) histology shows fat droplets in the capillaries and in the surrounding astrocytes. The patient suffered a mild head injury and a fractured femur and, later, became acutely ill with drowsiness and confusion about forty-eight hours after admission.

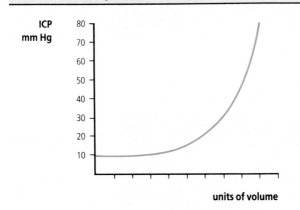

Relationship of intracranial pressure to increasing volume of intracranial contents

ICP mm Hg

units of volume

Fig. 17 Intracranial pressure/volume curve: fairly large changes in volume may occur chronically without substantial increase in pressure until a point is reached at which even small changes in volume do produce a substantial rise in pressure.

Transtentorial and tonsillar herniation

Slowly expanding intracranial haematomas and progressive brain swelling produce an increase in intracranial pressure but, initially, this is offset by reduction of the amount of CSF in the subarachnoid cisterns and probably by some reduction in cerebral blood flow. When the limits of these compensatory mechanisms are exceeded, a small rise in volume then produces a large rise in pressure.

The brain itself is incompressible, but it does shift at certain points, producing initially an effective reduction in intracranial volume. However, when the vertical component of the pressure volume curve is reached and severe shifts are produced, the consequences are generally very serious.

The effect of expanding masses above the tentorium is to displace cerebral tissue through the tentorial hiatus. Major tentorial herniation displaces the hippocampal gyrus downwards, compressing the oculomotor (III) nerve and, often, the posterior cerebral artery. The clinical effects are those of upper brain stem compression.

Unilateral supratentorial expanding masses cause lateral transtentorial herniation with displacement medially of the uncus, thus forcing the midbrain against the free edge of the tentorium. The usual clinical picture is that of ipsilateral oculomotor (III) nerve palsy, sometimes with ipsilateral compression of the posterior cerebral artery (and infarction in this arterial territory), and an ipsilateral hemiparesis due to the midbrain being forced against the tentorium on the opposite side (Kernohan's notch phenomenon). Unilateral supratentorial lesions may also produce horizontal displacement of the cingulate gyrus around the lower margin of the falx cerebri.

Supra- and infraorbital clots or swelling can also produce tonsillar herniation through the foramen magnum. Rapidly expanding masses within the posterior fossa often lead to acute respiratory arrest.

Exacerbation of the pressure differential between the supra- and infratentorial compartments, and between the infratentorial and spinal compartments, may lead to further brain herniation with irreversible effects on the functioning of the brain stem. For this reason, lumbar puncture is avoided in cases of head injury where mass effects have not been excluded.

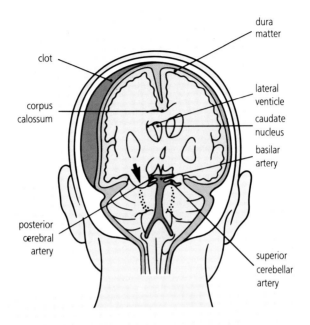

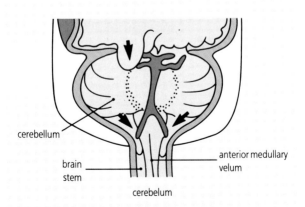

Fig. 18 Shift of brain tissue due to an expanding mass lesion within the cranial cavity. Such shifts may initially help to reduce the volume within the supra- or infratentorial compartments, but a continuing rise in pressure eventually produces irreversible damage.

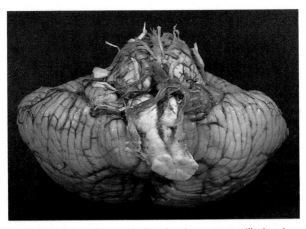

Fig. 19 Basal view of the cerebellum showing severe tonsillar herniation due to downward displacement from massively increased intracranial pressure.

IMMEDIATE ASSESSMENT AND TREATMENT

The immediate assessment and treatment of any head-injured patient requires attention to:
- Airway
- Breathing
- Circulation

Unconscious patients should have an airway inserted, if this can be tolerated, and be nursed semiprone unless a spinal injury is also strongly suspected. In cases of severe faciomaxillary injury or in which ventilation is inadequate, intubation and artificial ventilation may be immediately required. A rapid check is made for sources of continuing haemorrhage, particularly from the scalp and from arterial damage in the limbs, chest or abdomen. Hypovolaemia and hypotension necessitate intravenous infusion with replacement of blood loss. Fits should be aborted promptly with intravenous diazepam or intramuscular paraldehyde.

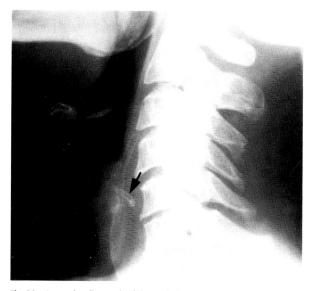

Fig. 20 Lateral radiograph of the neck showing a chicken bone (arrow) lodged in the throat. This illustration is included to emphasize the need to establish a clear airway and to remove food or debris from the back of the mouth.

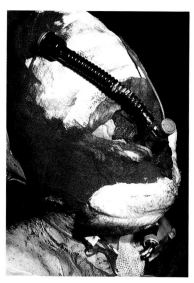

Fig. 21 This patient has severe facial and head injuries, and has both tracheostomy and endotracheal tubes in place(!), another demonstration of the importance of maintaining an airway.

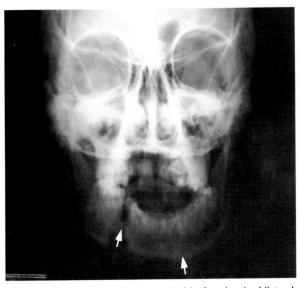

Fig. 22 Anteroposterior (AP) radiograph of the face showing bilateral mandibular fracture. Such cases are prone to obstructed airways due to the tongue rolling backwards and blocking the pharynx.

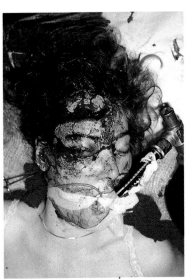

Fig. 23 Severe head injury resulting from multiple massive blows. The patient had lost a very substantial amount of blood from the scalp lacerations.

History

The clinical history is a most important factor in head trauma cases and is all too often overlooked. Head-injury management is one of anticipation based on recorded changes in the level of consciousness and neurological state at all stages of the illness from the time of onset. Eye-witness accounts of the accident are often of critical importance. It is essential to question witnesses or the ambulance crew as to the conscious level of the patient when first found and any subsequent deterioration or improvement. Ambulance crews can often also provide a good account of pupillary reaction soon after injury.

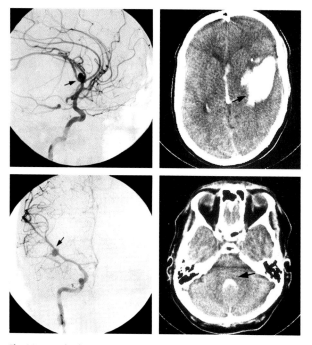

Fig. 24 Cerebral angiograms, lateral (upper left) and AP (lower left) views, and CT scans (right) showing rupture of a middle cerebral artery aneurysm (arrow) upwards into the temporal and parietal lobes. The resultant haematoma (arrow) then burst into the trigone of the lateral ventricle, causing severe intraventricular haemorrhage. This led to a road traffic accident (RTA). Fresh blood (arrow) was evident in the 4th ventricle (lower right).

When taking a clinical history, these are the questions to ask:

- What is the past medical history of the patient (diabetes, angina, hypertension)?
- Did the victim consume any drugs or alcohol?
- Could the accident have been caused by some other event, such as a subarachnoid haemorrhage or myocardial infarction?
- In children, could the injuries have been non-accidental?
- Was the victim wearing a seatbelt, crash helmet or riding hat?
- What were the time, place and details of the accident?
- What was the estimated blood loss at the site of the accident?
- What were the level of consciousness and pupillary reactions at the time of injury, and how have they changed?
- Has the patient had any fits?

Neurological examination

The key features of immediate neurological assessment are the level of consciousness and the presence of focal or lateral neurological signs. The vital signs of pulse, blood pressure and respiratory rate and rhythm should be noted on admission and clearly documented. When recording the level of consciousness, inexact phrases such as 'semiconscious' or 'semicomatose' should be avoided. Patients who are conscious may be alert, orientated and talking spontaneously or they may be disorientated, confused and thrashing about. With patients who are unconscious, the response to painful stimuli is recorded. This may be manifested as purposeful movements of the limbs, flexion, extension or a total absence of response.

The pupils are examined for size, symmetry and reaction to light, with differentiation between direct damage to the eye/optic (II) nerve and the oculomotor (III) nerve. Conjugate deviation or dysconjugate gaze of the eyes and the presence or absence of 'doll's-eye movements' are noted. Also to be considered are symmetry of limb movement or response to pain, reflex activity and other signs of cranial nerve deficit.

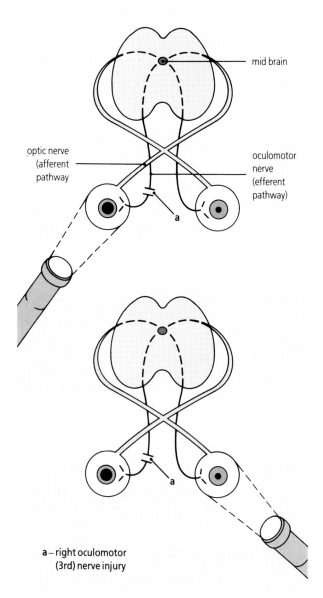

Fig. 25 Oculomotor (III) and optic (II) nerve damage: differential diagnosis.

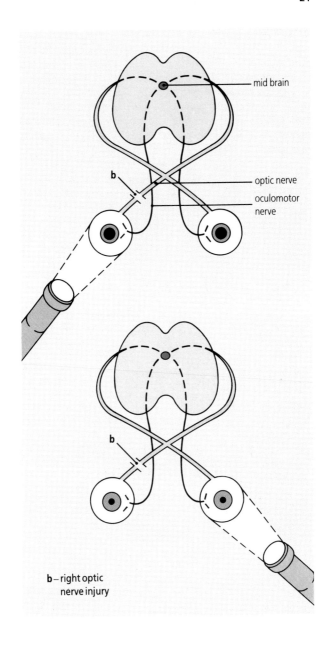

mid brain

b

optic nerve

oculomotor nerve

b – right optic nerve injury

Cases likely to involve spinal injury as well are often due to high-speed motorcycle crashes, diving into shallow water or falls from horses. Immobilization of the spine, with restricted movement and careful lifting, should be practised in all cases of suspected spinal injury until excluded, and suspected cervical injury may require immediate traction or halter fixation. The absence of movement and sensation below the level of suspected injury should be carefully recorded.

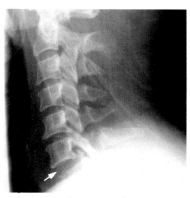

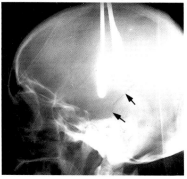

Fig. 26 A motorcycle accident victim: lateral radiograph of the neck (upper left) shows a fracture dislocation (arrow) at C6 and C7 which caused a pain response only when the upper limbs were flexed. The lateral radiograph of the skull (lower left) shows a linear temporo-parietal fracture (arrow) overlying branches of the middle meningeal artery. Traction calipers are also seen. The CT scan (right) shows a large extradural haematoma underlying the right-sided coup injury and fracture with extensive contrecoup contusion and haemorrhage within the left temporal lobe.

Although the spinal injury remains virtually total, the patient made a

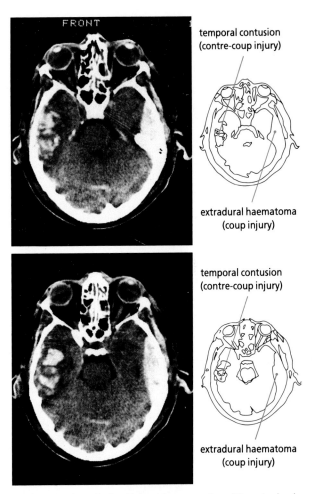

FRONT

temporal contusion
(contre-coup injury)

extradural haematoma
(coup injury)

temporal contusion
(contre-coup injury)

extradural haematoma
(coup injury)

good recovery from the head injury after evacuation of the extradural haematoma. As she is left-handed, her speech is unaffected by the left temporal damage.

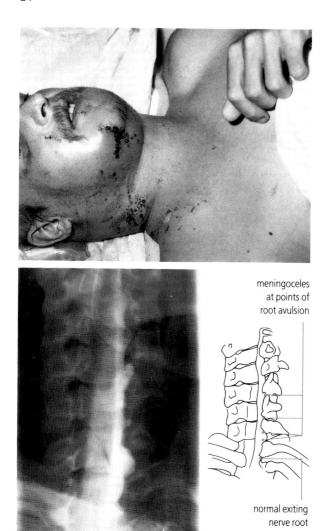

meningoceles
at points of
root avulsion

normal exiting
nerve root

Fig. 27 This motorcyclist, who was hit by a car, sustained head and facial injuries and an apparent spinal injury for which he was put in traction. Examination, however, revealed right facial and shoulder abrasions, a fractured clavicle (note the lump and line of skin discoloration over the shoulder) (upper) and a flail right arm, findings typical of an avulsion injury of the brachial plexus (lower). This is one film from a cervical myelogram (contrast is white) showing meningoceles at the points of root avulsion.

General examination

- Inspect and feel the entire scalp; fractures may be palpable beneath areas of boggy swelling.
- Extensive periorbital haematomas, bruising behind the ear (Battle's sign), bleeding from the ear and CSF rhinorrhoea or otorrhoea indicate fracture of the base of the skull.
- Look for compound depressed fractures of the vault with obvious leakage of CSF or cerebral tissue through the wound. Note the presence of foreign bodies.
- Note any injuries to the eye.
- Inspect the face for evidence of maxillary and mandibular fractures, particularly bilateral mandibular fractures.
- In infants, test the tension of the anterior fontanelle and feel for separation of cranial sutures. When non-accidental injury is supected, a general inspection should be made for limb and rib fractures and previous bruising and scars.
- Patients with suspected fractures of the spinal column should be treated as having such fractures until it is proved otherwise.
- Examine the chest for fractured sternum, flail segments, paradoxical respiration and evidence of pneumo- or haemothorax.
- Examine the abdomen for bruising (particularly seatbelt marks) over the liver and spleen, and for evidence of fluid within the peritoneal cavity. If in doubt, carry out peritoneal lavage.
- Inspect all limbs for evidence of long-bone fractures and immobilize as necessary.
- Ask for early assistance from appropriate surgical teams to help with suspected chest, abdominal or limb problems.
- It is essential that the cardiovascular and respiratory condition of the patient is as stable as possible before considering transfer to another centre or hospital for further assessment of injury.

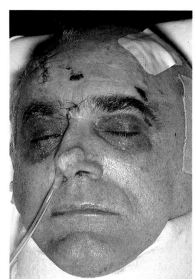

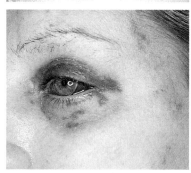

Fig. 28 Bilateral periorbital haematomas (upper) and complete subconjunctival haemorrhage and periorbital haematoma (lower) are indications of fracture of the base of the skull.

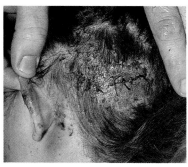

Fig. 29 Occipital lacerations are frequently missed because patients may be lying on their backs when first brought into casualty. This sutured laceration in the occipital region shows the characteristic boggy swelling and was overlying a site of fracture.

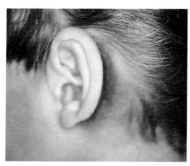

Fig. 30 Battle's sign: severe bruising behind the ear over the mastoid region implies a fracture of the base of the skull.

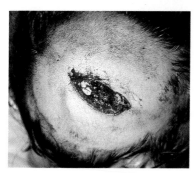

Fig. 31 Compound depressed fracture of the skull through which brain tissue and CSF is emerging. Hair has been shaved from around the wound and the scalp cleaned prior to inspection.

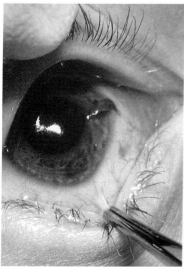

Fig. 32 Penetrating injury of the eye. The patient was unconscious on arrival and the injury was not discovered until the lids were passively opened and the eyes closely inspected.

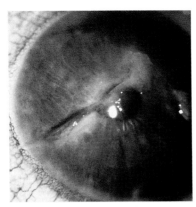

Fig. 33 Severe corneal laceration. All cases of head injury warrant careful inspection of the eyes during general examination.

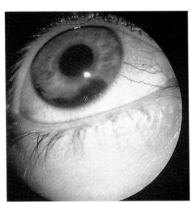

Fig. 34 Moderate hyphaema from being struck in the eye by a squash ball. His partner had earlier sustained a minor head injury due to a blow from a racquet.

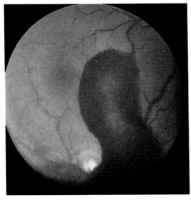

Fig. 35 Funduscopic view of the retina showing a large subhyaloid haemorrhage. This is virtually pathognomonic of subarachnoid haemorrhage and suggests that this event may have led to the trauma.

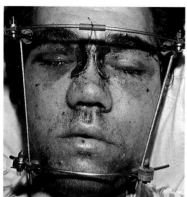

Fig. 36 Severe maxillo-facial injury with bilateral fractures of the mandible and of the base of the skull (note bilateral periorbital haematomas). Fixation bars were placed after reduction of the facial fractures and wiring of the mandible.

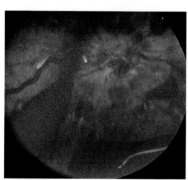

Fig. 37 Funduscopy showing severe multiple retinal haemorrhages in a child. This is seen in cases where the child has been severely shaken and raises suspicion of non-accidental injury.

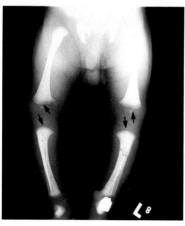

Fig. 38 Metaphyseal lucency (arrows) is a common feature of non-accidental injury and probably reflects the child's emotional and physical deprivation.

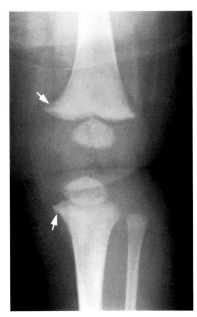

Fig. 39 Metaphyseal fractures, (arrows) whilst often very subtle, are a strong indication of non-accidental injury.

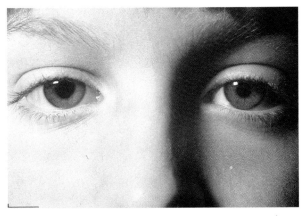

Fig. 40 This patient, who has a left Horner's syndrome (ptosis and miosis), suffered a minor head injury but also had a thoracic cord injury involving the T1 segment. He made a complete recovery.

PRELIMINARY INVESTIGATIONS

All patients with severe concussive head injuries must have adequate radiographs taken of the skull, chest and, when appropriate, cervical spine. Those with multiple injuries also require radiological examination of the appropriate limbs and abdomen.

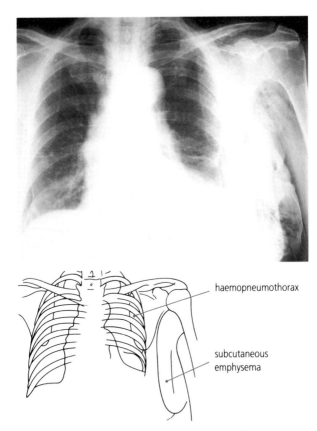

Fig. 41 Extensive subcutaneous emphysema obscures the haemopneumothorax caused by a penetrating chest injury.

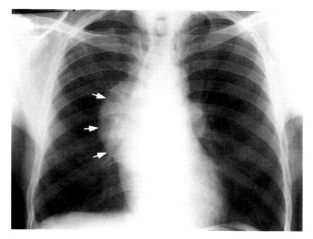

Fig. 42 In head-on collisions, the chest is thrust forward, subjecting the mediastinum and anterior chest wall to enormous deceleration forces. Veins and arteries are ruptured but, in this patient, the mediastinal mass is a haematoma (arrows) secondary to sternal fracture.

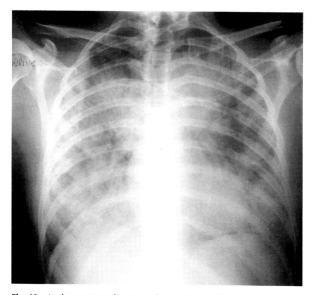

Fig. 43 In the context of acute and severe head injury, extensive consolidation of both lung fields but a heart of normal size implies pulmonary oedema of neurogenic origin.

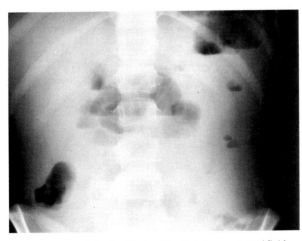

Fig. 44 An erect abdominal film in a 'silent' abdomen. Central fluid levels without gaseous distension suggests an ileus. In cases of 'pure' head injury, ileus is rarely long lasting.

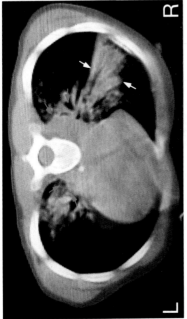

Fig. 45 This child was referred for a brain scan having been found unconscious after an R.T.A. The brans scan was normal but it was clear that the child was in respiratory distress and so a scan of the mediastinum was undertaken. The scan shows a pulmonary contusion (white arrows) and mediastinal widening (black arrows) caused by haematoma. Other scans (not shown) show that the trachea was undamaged.

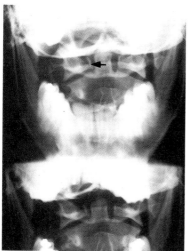

Fig. 46 As a result of an RTA and 'whiplash' flexion, there is a small fracture fragment (arrow) and slight misalignment of the odontoid peg (upper). CT scanning (lower) shows the avulsed fragment (white arrow) at the site of insertion of the transverse ligament. There is also a crush fracture (black arrow) of the arch of C1. This is an unstable fracture and requires active management.

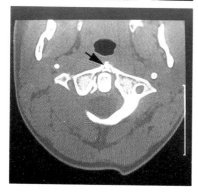

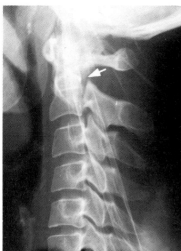

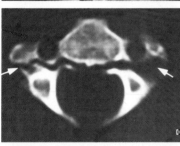

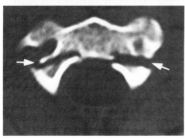

Fig. 47 As a result of severe whiplash from an RTA, the pedicles of C2 have been pulled off the vertebral body (arrow). The decision to use cervical traction is arrived at from plain radiographs (upper). The CT scans (lower) merely demonstrate the injury more elegantly.

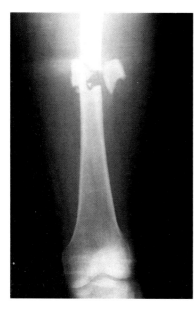

Fig. 48 An obvious fracture of the femur, but note the displaced muscular shadows due to a very large haematoma.

Radiography of the skull

Views of the skull include the anteroposterior, lateral and Towne's (thirty degrees from the brow upwards to clear the orbits and view the occipital region). If there is uncertainty concerning a depressed skull fracture, tangential views may be included.

The key features to examine on the skull radiograph are:

● Fractures

Do they overlie important structures which, if damaged, may cause bleeding or infection? Search should particularly be made for fractures over the middle meningeal artery, venous and air sinuses, and mastoid air cells. Do the fractures involve the base of the skull?

If depressed, are the fractures sufficiently deep to penetrate the dura mater and damage the underlying cortex?

- Is the pineal calcified?·If so, has it shifted laterally, indicating hemispheric displacement, or downwards, as in occasional cases of bilateral subdural haematomas?
- Are foreign bodies present?
- Is there air over the surface of the brain or within it? If so, there is a breach in the dura, usually associated with fracturing of the air sinuses. Are there fluid levels within the sinuses themselves?
- Are there any incidental findings suggesting pathology which may have contributed to the accident?

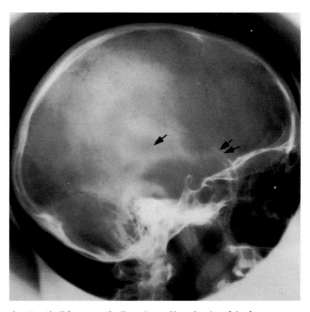

Fig. 49 Skull fracture. The linearity and low density of the fracture (white arrow) distinguish it from the normal vascular markings (black arrows).

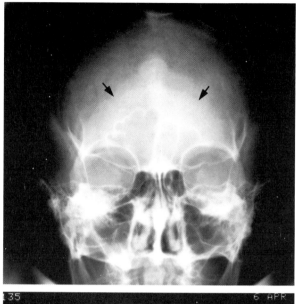

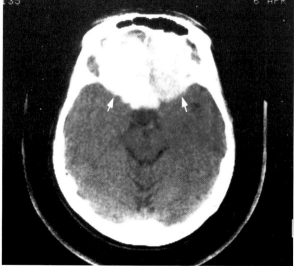

Fig. 50 PA radiograph (upper) and CT scan (lower) of an olfactory groove meningioma (arrowed) which contributed to head injury. The calcification within this tumour is clearly visible on the plain films, if it is looked for!

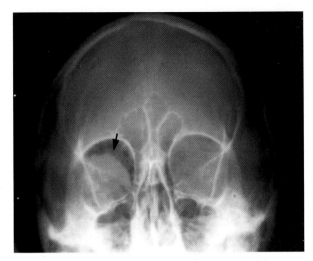

Fig. 51 Orbital emphysema following a direct blow to the right eye. The presence of gas (arrow) within the orbit indicates fracture into an adjacent air sinus. Opacity of the right ethmoid suggests the site. The bone fragments are too thin to be but rarely demonstrated on plain films; the fracture is inferred from changes in the soft tissues.

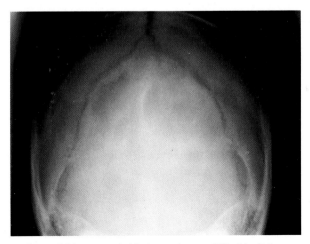

Fig. 52 In children, sutural widening can be very difficult to distinguish from the normal sutural appearance. This radiograph shows mild but definite sutural widening.

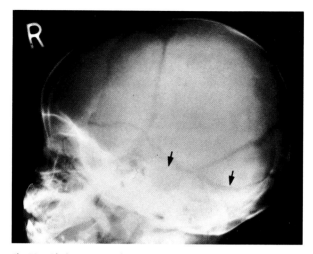

Fig. 53 Obvious severe, almost circumferential, skull fractures (arrow) are seen in this child brought into casualty by her anxious parent. The history given was of trivial trauma, but the discrepancy between the history and radiographic findings is a classical feature of non-accidental injury.

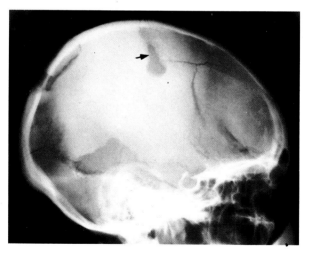

Fig. 54 This depressed 'slot' fracture (arrow) with multiple direct and tangential fractures is the result of a low-velocity high-force injury from axe blows.

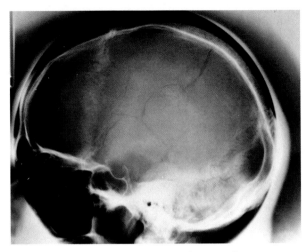

Fig. 55 This 'crazy-paving' pattern of skull fracture reflects an enormous transference of energy. The patient had experienced a glancing blow from a high-velocity bullet. A less tangential trajectory would have been lethal.

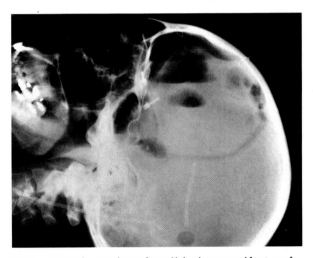

Fig. 56 Aerocoele secondary to frontal lobe damage and fracture of the cribriform plate. The patient was stabbed in the eye by an umbrella spike. The injury also produced a traumatic arterial aneurysm which has been clipped. A ventriculoperitoneal shunt is in place.

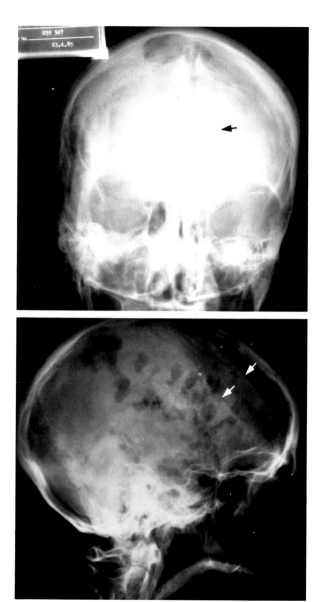

Fig. 57 This PA radiograph (upper left) shows a fracture (arrow) running into the frontal sinus, thus allowing direct communication to the outside. The lateral view (lower left) and CT scans (right) reveal almost

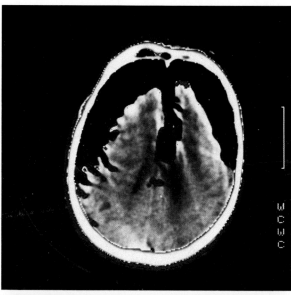

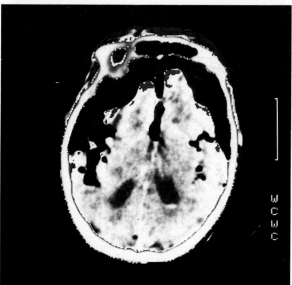

unbelievable quantities of intracranial air and fluid levels (arrow). Surprisingly, the patient was confused but only mildly drowsy.

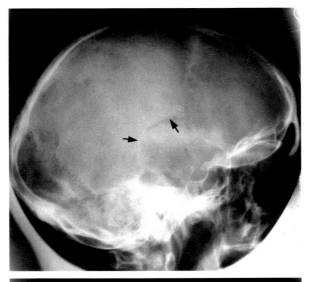

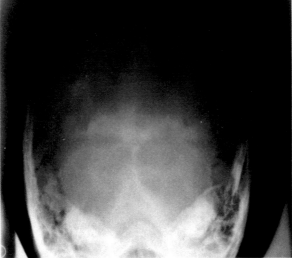

Fig. 58 Lateral radiograph (upper) of a patient who was hit on the side of the head with a heavy metal object. Note how the dark line becomes a white line (arrowed), a classical appearance of a depressed fracture caused by overriding of the fracture fragment. Confirmation is by a Towne's view (lower), which shows the fracture fragment (arrowed). However, this fracture was missed by the casualty officer!

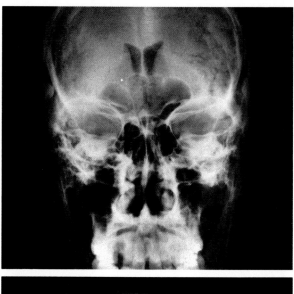

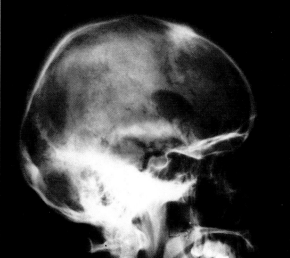

Fig. 59 PA (upper) and lateral (lower) radiographs showing air within the ventricles which entered via a traumatic cisternal puncture; the victim had been stabbed in the neck.

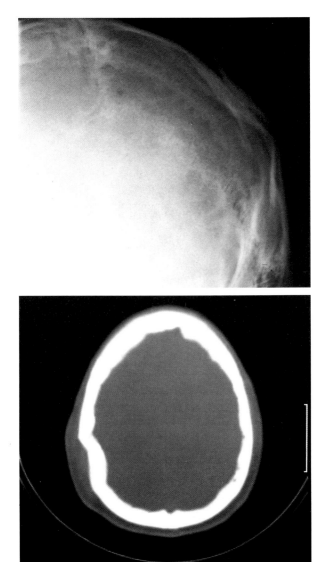

Fig. 60 Depressed fractures may be entirely invisible on straight radiography. If these fractures are suspected, radiographers should provide tangential views (upper) which do demonstrate these lesions. They are easily demonstrated on CT scanning (lower).

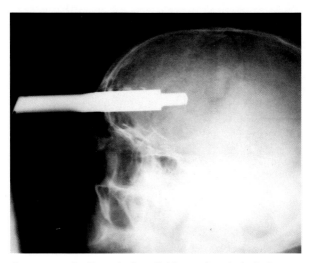

Fig. 61 Lateral radiograph of a scaffolding worker who looked up to see a bolt falling towards him; it pierced his left frontal lobe. A helmet would have spared him such a devastating injury.

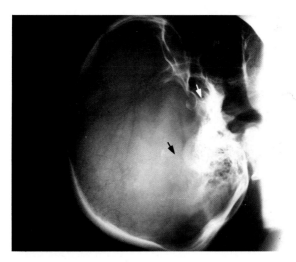

Fig. 62 This patient was bleeding from the ear. Radiography shows a linear fracture in the posterior temporal region (black arrow). The clinical question is whether this is a simple fracture of the vault or does it extend across the base of the skull. The presence of fluid in the sphenoid (white arrow) indicates the latter.

EARLY MANAGEMENT

Adult patients with minor or moderate concussive head injuries, no focal neurology nor skull fracture are most likely to make a good recovery. Usually their only requirement is simple observation. However, children may develop extradural haematoma even in the absence of skull fractures. Care must also be taken not to overlook serious injury in habitual drunks who frequent Casualty Departments. The general aim is to prevent or treat secondary brain surgery.

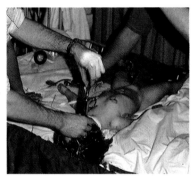

Fig. 63 This child had a massive extradural haematoma with sudden deterioration but was very late arriving at the hospital. Such futile attempts to evacuate the haematoma in casualty should be preventable.

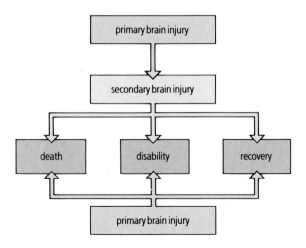

Fig. 64 Primary brain injury may be followed directly or indirectly by death, disability or recovery.

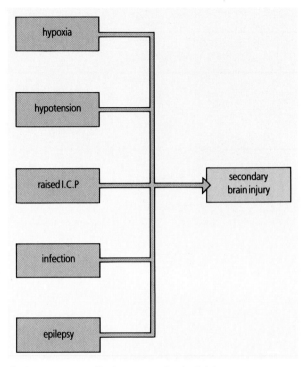

Fig. 65 Factors contributing to secondary brain injury.

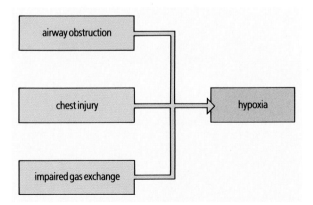

Fig. 66 Factors in head-injured patients which may contribute to hypoxia which, in turn, leads to further brain damage.

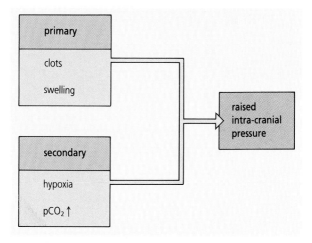

Fig. 67 Potential causes of raised intracranial pressure following head injury.

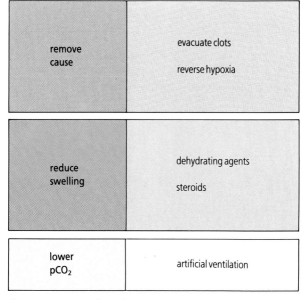

Fig. 68 Treatment of raised intracranial pressure.

Glasgow coma scale		
eyes open	spontaneously	to pain
	to speech	none
best verbal response	orientated	incomprehensible sounds
	confused	none
	inappropriate words	
best motor response	obey commands	extension to pain
	localise pain	none
	flexion to pain	

NEUROLOGICAL OBSERVATION CHART — HOSPITAL

Surname: First Name: Date of Birth Sex Unit Number Consultant/s

			DATE
Frequency of recordings			TIME

COMA SCALE

eyes open	spontaneously		eyes closed by swelling – C
	to speech		
	to pain		
	none		
best verbal response	orientated		endotracheal tube or tracheostomy – T
	confused		
	inappropriate words		
	incomprehensible sounds		
	none		
best motor response	obey commands		usually record the best arm response
	localise pain		
	flexion pain		
	extension to pain		
	none		

written comments – see over

blood pressure and pulse rate

240 220 200 180 160 140 120 100 80 60 40

pupil scale (mm) 1 2 3 4 5 6 7 8

respiration 20

temperature °C 41 40 39 38 37 36 35 34 33 32 31

PUPILS

right	size		+ reacts
	reaction		– no reaction
left	size		c eyes closed by swelling
	reaction		

LIMB MOVEMENT

ARMS

normal power		
mild weakness		
severe weakness		
spastic flexion		
extension		
no response		

LEGS

normal power		
mild weakness		
severe weakness		
extension		
no response		

record right (R) and left (L) separately if there is a difference between the two sides

Fig. 69 a The Glasgow coma scale (upper) and (lower) incorporated into an intensive care/neurological chart for clear recording of the patient's progress on the ward.

52

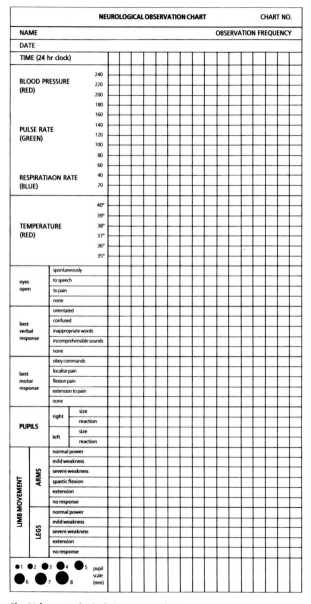

Fig. 69 b Neurological observation chart.

Clinical assessment and the results of the preliminary radiological investigations dictate further management and prompt the following questions:

- Has the patient deteriorated or remained stable from the time of injury? If stable, are there adverse clinical or radiological factors which suggest deterioration may occur?
- Is there evidence of increasing intracranial pressure (decreasing level of consciousness) or of developing neurological signs (progressive focal pathology)? If so, how rapidly are these progressing?
- Has the patient had epileptic fits following injury?

Management now depends upon judging whether a patient has progressive but potentially reversible intracranial pathology and upon the speed of deterioration, if any. Patients with closed head injuries who are improving, and those in a stable condition with no risk factors, may simply require observation on the ward. Their neurological state is recorded carefully on a detailed chart incorporating the Glasgow coma scale, which is easy for subsequent observers to interpret.

Patients who are rendered deeply unconscious from the time of the accident but whose condition has deteriorated no further on admission are probably suffering from primary brain injury. They also may simply require careful observation whilst their other injuries are treated and their general condition stabilized.

Raised intracranial pressure from brain swelling and acute subdural haematoma (which is most often associated with severe primary brain injury) is generally difficult to treat and not always reversible. From the practical point of view, the most important pathology to exclude is acute extradural haematoma. This potentially lethal condition is completely reversible if it is recognized early and the clot evacuated promptly.

FURTHER INVESTIGATIONS AND MANAGEMENT

Computerized tomographic (CT) scanning

The CT scan is an integral part of modern management of head-injured patients. Scanners with short scan times allow reasonable pictures even of restless patients. However, most District General Hospitals in the United Kingdom do not have access to CT scanning facilities. A decision must be made, depending on the patient's condition, whether immediate surgical treatment is necessary or whether transfer to a more specialized unit is required.

The scan can exclude or confirm and localize intracranial haematomas, demonstrate swelling and diffuse injury of the brain, clarify the extent of damage distant from the site of direct injury and expose the presence of hydrocephalus.

Indications for neurosurgical assessment

- Coma (no eye-opening, recognizable speech or motor response to commands) persisting for more than six hours after injury;
- Obvious deterioration of neurological state or level of consciousness;
- Failure to achieve full consciousness and orientation within twenty-four hours after admission;
- Presence of focal neurological signs, including those from the time of injury;
- Post-traumatic generalized or focal epilepsy;
- Compound depressed fractures;
- Suspected intracranial haematoma.

Not all patients who have failed to recover fully within twenty-four hours of injury require transfer; the necessity or otherwise should be discussed with the neurosurgical team.

Unconscious patients being transferred to distant scanning or neurosurgical facilities should be accompanied by an anaesthetist. If there is a suspected risk of respiratory arrest or embarrassment, it is safer to intubate and ventilate the patient prior to transfer, even though this may make neurological assessment more difficult.

- All patients must be adequately resuscitated and sources of major bleeding controlled before transfer.

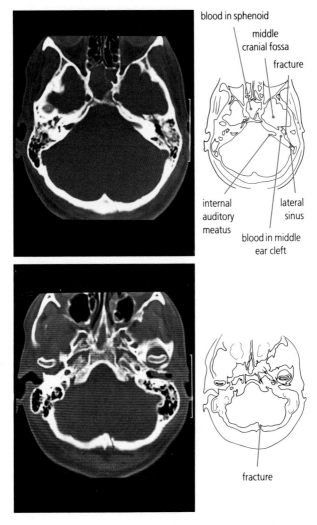

blood in sphenoid

middle cranial fossa

fracture

internal auditory meatus

lateral sinus

blood in middle ear cleft

fracture

Fig. 70 Fracture of the base of the skull is often impossible to detect radiographically, but requires CT scanning through the base of the skull. This fracture has traversed the petrous bone at the level of the middle ear cleft and extended across the floor of the middle cranial fossa to involve the wall of the sphenoid air sinus (which is full of blood) and the carotid canal. There is also a midline fracture of the occipital bone. This is a compound injury and its severity is evidenced by its involvement of important structures.

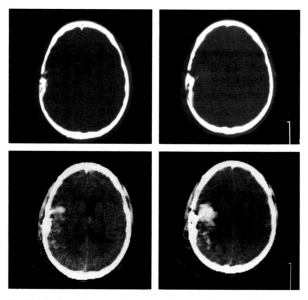

Fig. 71 In these CT scans of a depressed splinter fracture, the bone window (upper) shows the bony splinters while the soft tissue window (lower) shows the associated contusion.

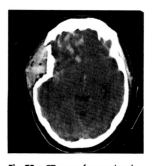

Fig. 72 CT scan of a massive depressed fracture with associated left frontal lobe contusion. Note the air bubbles in the brain and soft tissue of the scalp.

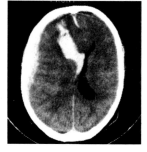

Fig. 73 CT scan of a fresh subdural haematoma associated with a fracture of the skull. interestingly, the injury has also split the left frontal lobe and extends into the frontal horn. The subdural haematoma extends along the falx cerebri.

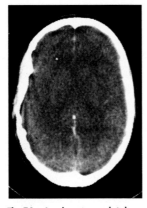

Fig. 74 An almost completely featureless CT scan as seen here reflects gross cerebral oedema and disorganization; this is almost always fatal.

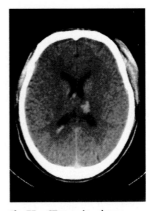

Fig. 75 CT scanning shows petechial haemorrhages, which frequently arise close to the walls of the ventricles (as seen here) and at the grey/white matter interfaces.

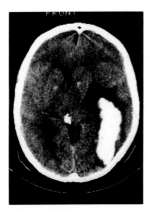

Fig. 76 CT scans of a large parieto-occipital haematoma. The effect of this lesion is a severe shift of the midline pineal (arrow) to the left.

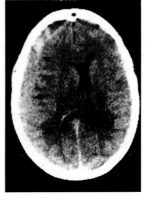

Fig. 77 There is a point at which the density of a subdural haematoma is equal to that of the brain (isodensity). Modern scanners, capable of resolving the grey/white interfaces (arrows), clearly demonstrate the resultant displacement of the cerebral surface.

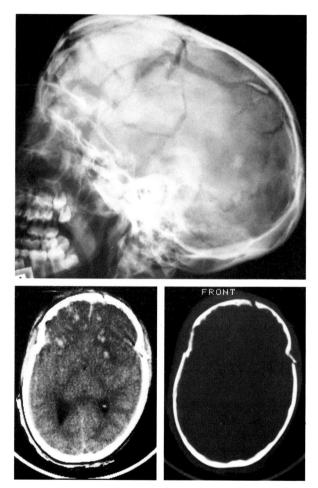

Fig. 78 Lateral radiograph (upper) and CT scans (lower) of a severe head injury that has shattered the skull. Note the numerous petechial haemorrhages in the frontal region.

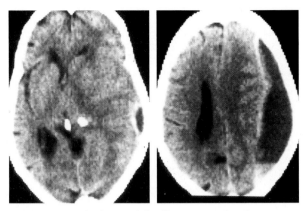

Fig. 79 CT scans of a chronic subdural haematoma. There is an enormous amount of shift on the low scanning cut (left) and only the edge of the haematoma is visible. At higher cuts (right), more of the haematoma can be seen with cellular debris in its posterior aspect.

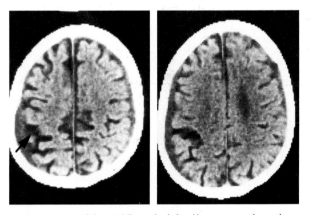

Fig. 80 CT scans of chronic bilateral subdural haematomas (arrow). Note the atrophied and shrunken appearance of the brain in this alcoholic patient; let this be a warning!

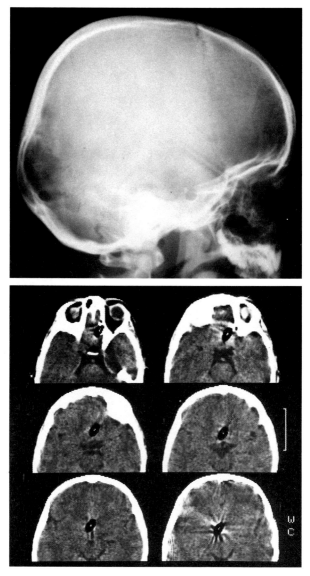

Fig. 81 Lateral radiograph (upper) and a series of CT scans (lower) of a child who fell on a pencil which penetrated the orbit. The wood shows low density on both types of imaging (black areas on CT scans). Amazingly, no important cerebral structure was damaged.

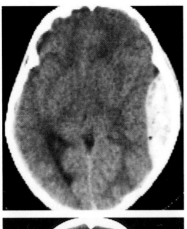

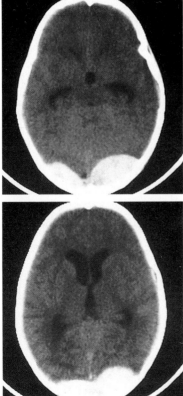

Fig. 82 CT scans of extradural haematomas. The classical biconvex shape (upper) is due to its being under high pressure and bounded by the adherent dura. The effect of mass from the occipital extradural haematomas (middle & lower) is hydrocephalus from compression of the aquaduct.

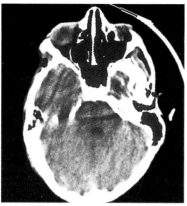

Fig. 83 CT scans showing the normal appearance of the brain stem and the fourth ventricle (upper); two days later (middle & lower), these structures were obliterated by severe oedema in the posterior fossa. Low scanning cuts show the foramen magnum filled with posterior fossa contents, indicating coning. The patient died.

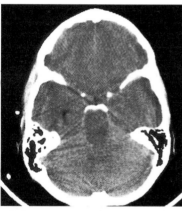

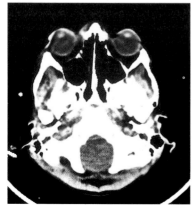

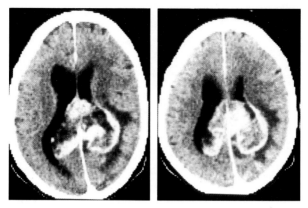

Fig. 84 CT scans of an irregular tumour extending on both sides of the midline in the corpus callosum. These are the classical appearances of a 'butterfly' glioma. The patient was involved in an RTA which may have been caused by a fit.

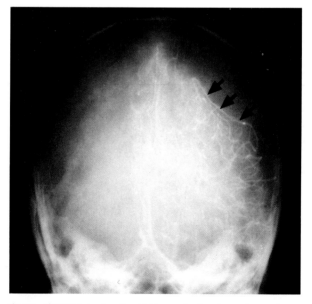

Fig. 85 If CT scanning is not available, cerebral angiography may be used to demonstrate the underlying pathology in cases of head injury. In this angiogram of an extradural haematoma, displacement of vessels (arrows) away from the inner table of the skull is clearly seen.

Surgical management

Acute extradural haematoma

Acute extradural haematoma (EDH) is most often associated with fracture of the skull over one or more branches of the middle meningeal artery. It may mimic 'primary brain injury' with profound or rapidly progressive loss of consciousness and fixed neurological deficit from the time of trauma; however, the classical sequence of events is:

> The patient is initially knocked out by a blow to the head. A small clot forms in the extradural space due to rupture of one of the middle meningeal vessels. If the injury is not too severe, the patient may subsequently improve to the extent of full alertness and speech (the lucid interval). At this time the clot is enlarging, thus pushing aside more dura from the inner surface of the skull and causing further bleeding. Eventually the entire cerebral hemisphere becomes displaced medially, causing compression of the oculomotor (III) nerve and brain stem, and a rise in intracranial pressure. The classical signs are those of a secondary deterioration in the level of consciousness, bradycardia and hypertension, with a dilated non-reacting pupil and ipsilateral or sometimes contralateral hemiparesis.

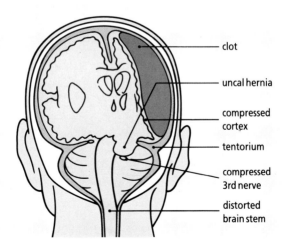

Fig. 86 The effects of an expanding mass (extradural haematoma) including brain shift and tentorial herniation.

Patients presenting with this history and some or all of these clinical features require very prompt attention to exclude extradural haematoma. If the deterioration is gradual, the patient may be given a diuretic agent (intravenous frusemide or twenty percent mannitol) and transferred to the nearest neurosurgical unit, accompanied by an anaesthetist.

If the deterioration is rapid, a long journey by ambulance should not be undertaken. If CT scanning is available in the hospital and time permits, the exact site of the clot should be determined.

If the patient is obviously coning or has respiratory irregularity, he should be taken immediately to the operating theatre. After the head is shaved, a burr-hole is placed over the site of fracture as indicated on radiography. If an extradural haematoma is found, the burr-hole is enlarged to provide a generous craniectomy and allow evacuation of the haematoma, thus relieving pressure on the brain stem. Bleeding from the exposed area may be controlled by applying gentle pressure over a pack. The patient, still under assisted ventilation, is then transferred immediately to the nearest neurosurgical centre whilst any blood losses are continuously being replaced.

If there is no fracture in a suspected case of EDH, after the head is shaved, a burr-hole should be made directly above the zygoma on the side of the dilated pupil. A second burr-hole is made in the frontal region at the hairline at the level of the normal position of the pupil in forward gaze. A third burr-hole is made above and behind the ear in the parietal region. If a clot is found, a craniectomy is performed around the appropriate burr-holes.

If no haematoma is found either underlying a fracture or under the initial three burr-holes, a further three similarly placed burr-holes should be made on the opposite side. Only then can an extradural haematoma be completely excluded.

Patients explored for EDH by a surgeon inexperienced in dealing with these conditions should, after surgery, be transferred immediately to the nearest neurosurgical centre.

Formal neurosurgical exploration for extradural haematoma is by craniotomy. Burr-holes or a craniectomy from previous exploration can be readily converted to a craniotomy exposure if the former are correctly sited.

Early management of extradural haematoma also includes prophylactic anticonvulsant medication, usually with phenytoin.

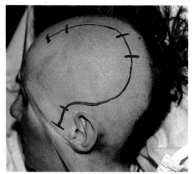

Fig. 87 Scalp incision for a craniotomy to remove a typical frontotemporal extradural haematoma. The burr-hole sites for exploration for haematoma are also indicated. Note the presence of Battle's sign.

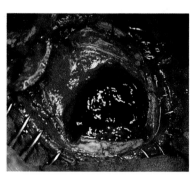

Fig. 88 The bone flap has been pulled aside, revealing a small extradural haematoma.

Acute subdural haematoma

This is often clinically indistinguishable from primary head injury and is usually diagnosed on CT scanning. There is frequently diffuse accompanying cerebral swelling and patients are often in a critical neurological condition. The solid clot forms a thin layer over the brain surface and is evacuated through a craniotomy, avoiding a wide incision in the dura which may be impossible to close.

Chronic subdural haematoma

These liquid haematomas are usually diagnosed a few weeks

after injury on the basis of a fluctuating level of consciousness, headaches or the slow development of diffuse lateralized neurological signs. Evacuation is usually through frontal and parietal burr-holes at the sites described earlier for extradural haematoma.

Depressed skull fracture
The depressed segments may be elevated through a burr-hole adjacent to the skull depression; at that time, the dura can be inspected for lacerations. Large clean bone fragments may be replaced over the dura to avoid the need for extensive cranioplasty.

Compound vault fractures without depression
These require exploration sufficient to confirm that there is no depression of the skull and no penetration by foreign bodies. The scalp is sutured in two layers as is usual. Antibiotic medication is not necessary in these cases.

Prophylactic antibiotic cover, such as ampicillin and flucloxacillin, is usually given in cases where radiography shows linear fractures through mastoid air cells and sinuses, air within the cranial cavity or CSF otorrhoea or rhinorrhoea is present. Virtually all cases of CSF otorrhoea cease spontaneously and at least seventy percent of cases of CSF rhinorrhoea cease within seven days.

Compound depressed skull fractures
Obvious compound depressed fractures of the vault or depressed fractures through the air sinuses require adequate neurosurgical exploration within a period of eight to twelve hours. The early management of compound depressed fractures includes cleaning and shaving the scalp around the fracture/laceration, placing a dry dressing over the affected area and applying a head bandage. If there is an excess of dirt or foreign body superficially in the scalp lesions, the latter must be cleaned first; if there is excessive bleeding from the lesion, the wound needs closing temporarily. The patient should be placed on prophylactic anticonvulsant and antibiotic medication. No attempt should be made to remove obvious deep penetrating foreign bodies; these should only be removed when formal craniotomy can be safely performed.

Compound depressed skull fractures must always be explored thoroughly, either by using a formal scalp flap or by extending the scalp laceration. It is essential to remove all fragments of dead bone, foreign bodies, dirt and non-viable brain, and to obtain good haemostasis. When the dura has been torn, it should be repaired if possible. Patients require prophylactic anticonvulsants and antibiotics unless there has been no dural laceration. Missile injuries to the head usually require extensive debridement.

Repair of orbital margins and other bony contours

This is sometimes undertaken as a primary repair at the same time as other skull fractures are being treated, but may be combined with late surgery in cases of severe facial injury and CSF rhinorrhoea.

Cranioplasty

Large craniectomy sites may require replacement surgery. Wherever possible, the patient's own bone is used but, in cases of severe extensive comminuted or dirty skull fractures, this may not be possible. The usual materials for cranioplasty are acrylic cement with or without titanium mesh, titanium plates and split calvarial grafts.

Insertion of intracranial pressure monitors

This can be of great value in the management of primary brain injury with cerebral swelling. Either a subdural catheter inserted through a burr-hole or an epidural monitoring system is connected through a pressure transducer to recording apparatus. Intracranial pressure can then be monitored continuously and diuretic therapy administered to reduce intracranial pressure during its elevated phases, thus avoiding excessive dehydration or fluid overload.

Hydrocephalus

Ventricular drainage or ventriculoperitoneal shunting is sometimes necessary in cases of post-traumatic hydrocephalus

Persistent CSF fistulas

Virtually all cases of traumatic CSF otorrhoea cease spontaneously. CSF rhinorrhoea persisting for more than about ten days may require surgical correction by dural repair.

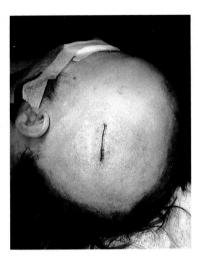

Fig. 89 Scalp laceration overlying a compound depressed fracture. Note how the head has been shaved in preparation for exploration.

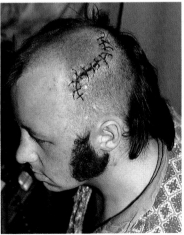

Fig. 90 An S-shaped extension above the laceration to facilitate elevation of the fracture (same patient as in Fig. 89).

Medical management

General measures

At any stage in the post-traumatic period, deterioration in the level of consciousness or overall neurological state requires prompt investigation and treatment of expanding intracranial lesions. The other main requirements of medical care include control of fits, treatment of infection, adequate care and control of respiratory dysfunction, and general care of the unconscious patient.

Unconscious patients should be regularly turned from side to side to prevent pressure sores. The airway must be protected and the aspiration of bronchial secretions prevented in those with poor cough or gag reflexes; if necessary, a cuffed endotracheal tube can be inserted or tracheostomy performed.

Except in cases of CSF rhinorrhoea, a nasogastric tube is inserted and, in the acute phase, the stomach kept empty to avoid regurgitation. Thereafter, most patients suffering solely from head injury absorb fluid well through the gut and may be fed in this manner. Blood or other major fluid loss and electrolyte imbalance are corrected by intravenous infusion, avoiding continuous replacement with normal saline.

Medication

Most drugs may be administered via the nasogastric tube. This is particularly important in the case of phenytoin, which is irregularly absorbed intramuscularly and should be given intravenously only with great caution to avoid cardiac dysrhythmias.

If intracranial haematoma has been excluded and the neurological deterioration is due to progressive brain swelling, intravenous frusemide (10-40mg) or twenty percent mannitol (200ml over 20 min) may be administered. The dose and frequency may be judged by improvement in level of consciousness, by pupillary size or by recording the intracranial pressure directly. To maintain cerebral perfusion pressure, it is preferable to avoid prolonged episodes of hypotension.

Other agents often used are:

Anticonvulsant agents: in cases of extradural haematoma, compound depressed fractures, severe cerebral contusion and intracerebral haemorrhage, and immediate post-traumatic or preexisting epilepsy.

Antibiotics: may be used for prophylaxis in cases of compound depressed skull fractures with penetration of the dura, and for CSF otorrhoea and rhinorrhoea.

Antacid preparations: may be delivered via a nasogastric tube to prevent acute gastric erosion, which is sometimes seen in severely head-injured patients.

Analgesia: patients with other severe injuries may require large amounts of analgesics. If opiates are used, these patients must be assessed carefully and frequently by experienced staff. In cases of pure head injury, it is preferable to avoid the major opiates, which depress respiration and level of consciousness and mask neurological signs. Codeine phosphate or DF118 are the most commonly used analgesics in these cases.

Sedatives: occasionally, patients who are confused and restless require sedation. Small doses of chlorpromazine may be used but only if body temperature is carefully controlled and no hypotension results.

Antidiuretics: patients with basal skull fractures may develop diabetes insipidus and thus require antidiuretic therapy.

There is little evidence that steroids play a significant role in reducing cerebral oedema in head injury; their routine use is not advocated. Hyperventilation as a means of reducing intracranial pressure, and barbiturates and hypothermia to 'protect' the brain by reducing metabolic requirements are probably of very limited value.

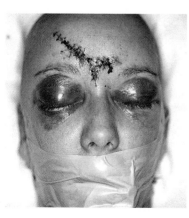

Fig. 91 Extension of a right frontal laceration to facilitate repair of a compound depressed fracture of the anterior wall of the frontal sinus.

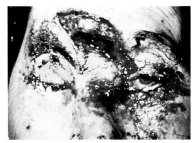

Fig. 92 These severe facial lacerations and abrasions with fracture into the frontal air sinus are best dealt with by a combination of neuro-surgical and plastic surgery teams.

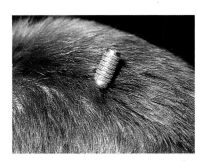

Fig. 93 This partially embedded dart in the head was thrown at a football match. Foreign objects causing severe injuries (see also Fig. 61) should not be removed in the casualty depart-ment but in the operating theatre.

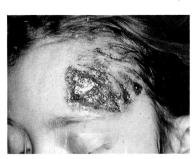

Fig. 94 Extensive scalp abrasions in a child. These abrasions often contain large amounts of road dirt or other foreign material and require thorough cleaning and scrubbing under general anaesthetic to minimize cosmetic deformity.

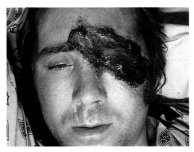

Fig. 95 Severe road burns to the face. These are best treated in con-junction with a plastic surgeon.

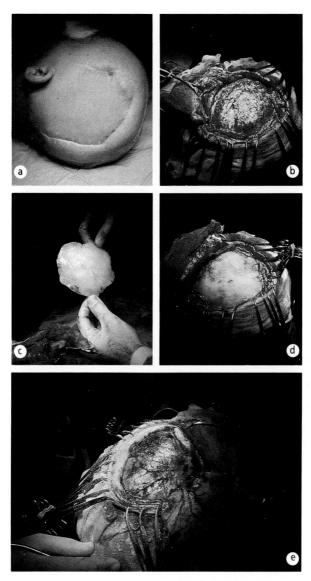

Fig. 96 Acrylic cranioplasty: (a) previous craniotomy scar and skull defect; (b) exposure of the dura and edges of the bony defect; (c) the specially made acrylic plate; (d) acrylic plate insertion; (e) suturing the plate to the cranial margin.

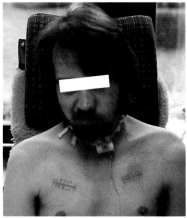

Fig. 97 This patient sustained a severe lower brain stem and upper cervical injury from which he made a partial recovery. He required constant ventilation but was ultimately treated by the insertion of bilateral phrenic pacing devices (note the healed incisions in the chest). The devices maintain ventilation and allow a reasonable degree of independence.

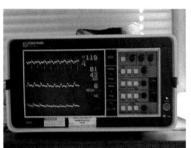

Fig. 98 This is used to continuously record the patients intracranial pressure, and when connected to a digital reader, also give a clear, simultaneous indication of blood pressure and pulse.

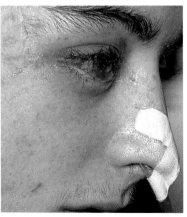

Fig. 99 Eye care is important in patients who remain unconscious for long periods of time to prevent drying of the conjunctiva and corneal abrasions, which occurred in this patient. Care must be taken with nasal tubes and tapes not to erode skin and cartilage.

COMPLICATIONS

The major early complications following head injury are raised intracranial pressure from brain swelling or intracranial haematoma, and a cycle of secondary deterioration related to hypoxia and hypotension.

Other short-term complications include:

Meningitis and intracranial abscess or empyema.

These are most likely to occur in patients with major compound depressed fractures or fractures through the air sinuses. An established meningitis should be treated with high-dose intravenous antibiotics. Cerebral abscess must be treated by drainage or excision and intravenous antibiotic therapy.

Epilepsy.

All fits should be treated promptly, using intravenous diazepam initially. If a single dose is ineffective, intramuscular paraldehyde is necessary. If generalized convulsions continue, the patient may require a thiopentone infusion with artificial ventilation and careful control of blood pressure. When paralyzing agents are used, EEG monitoring may exclude unrecognized continuing seizures. Prophylactic anticonvulsants are usually given to high-risk patients.

Patients at greatest risk of delayed post-traumatic epilepsy are those who have had fits immediately after injury, those with intracranial haematoma, those with compound depressed skull fractures and those with a post-traumatic amnesia of more than twenty-four hours. Various combinations of these risk factors may increase the likelihood of late-onset epilepsy to over sixty percent.

Hyperpyrexia.

Patients with diffuse brain injury and brain stem dysfunction may exhibit hyperpyrexia and swings in blood pressure and pulse rate. Hyperpyrexia is treated by tepid sponging and by chlorpromazine, provided that the blood pressure and temperature do not drop profoundly.

Long-term complications include chest and intracranial infection, pressure sores, fixed contractures of limbs and joints, and weight loss through muscle wasting and sometimes through poor dietary control. Hydrocephalus, chronic subdural haematoma, post-traumatic epilepsy and skull defects have already been described. An important but rare complication is caroticocavernous fistula.

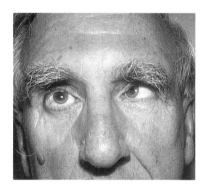

Fig. 100 Right abducens (VI) nerve palsy following head injury. This frequently is of no localizing value neurologically.

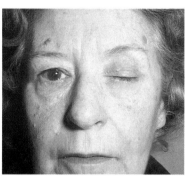

Fig. 101 Left oculomotor (III) nerve palsy following head injury. Note the ptosis (upper) and failure of upward gaze and adduction (lower).

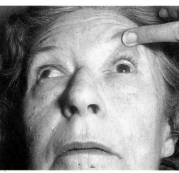

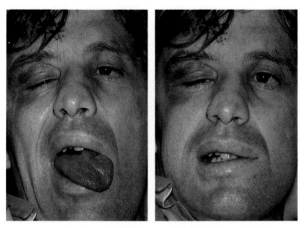

Fig. 102 Massive fracturing of the base of the skull has resulted in (left) left trigeminal (V), facial (VII), vestibulocochlear (VIII) and hypoglossal (XII), and (right) right oculomotor (III) nerve palsies.

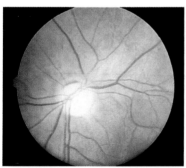

Fig. 103 Funduscopy shows consecutive optic atrophy due to optic nerve damage following head injury.

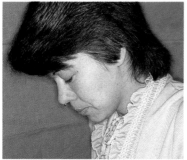

Fig. 104 CSF rhinorrhoea. By bending forwards and performing a Valsalva manoeuvre, CSF can be seen leaking from the nose.

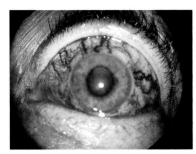

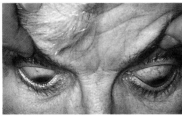

Fig. 105 This eye is proptosed and suffused with prominent vessels (upper) due to a post-traumatic carotico-cavernous fistula. There is a pulsating exophthalmos (lower).

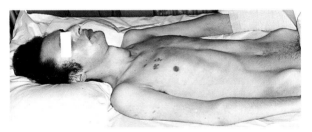

Fig. 106 Profound weight loss following severe generalized primary head injury. Great care must be taken during nursing to avoid pressure sores and fixed contraction deformities.

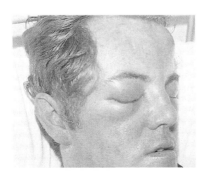

Fig. 107 Pott's puffy tumour in severe frontal osteomyelitis. The patient had a fever with a soft fluctuant tender swelling over the left frontal region; the underlying pathology was frontal sinusitis. Such infection can develop from skull fractures into the sinuses.

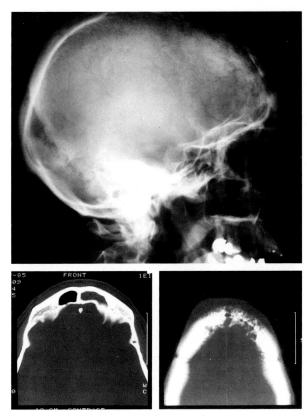

Fig. 108 Lateral radiograph (upper) and CT scan (lower) of osteomyelitis of the frontal bone. Note the extensive destruction and opaque frontal sinus. The infective organism is almost always Streptococcus milleri.

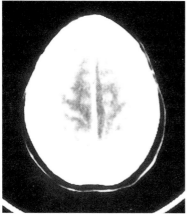

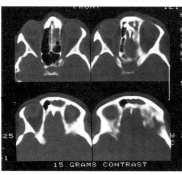

Fig. 109 CT scan of a subdural empyema. The clinical condition is usually much more severe than the scan suggests, as the changes are very subtle. Note the parafalcine collections of pus (upper), seen as a dark strip parallel to the enhanced (white) falx cerebri, and associated frontal and ethmoidal sinusitis (lower).

BRAIN DEATH

Two forms of irreversible brain damage occur. The first is when there is no cortical function. A patient in this state may survive for many years in a vegetative state, sometimes without artificial ventilation. The other form is when the brain stem ceases to function. In these cases, the heart stops beating within, at most, a few days of withdrawal of artificial ventilation.

To avoid the often distressing consequences of prolonged ventilation of an already brain-dead patient, it is important to be able to identify correctly the point at which brain-stem death has occurred. Guidelines have been laid down for conducting tests for brain-stem function and for making the diagnosis of brain death. These include:

- There is no evidence that brain-stem depression is related to hypothermia, metabolic factors or depressant drug treatment.
- The primary diagnosis (head injury) is known.
- There is no spontaneous respiration (and muscle relaxants are not being used) when the arterial pCO_2 is greater than 6.65 kPa
- The patient exhibits no response to painful stimuli.
- The pupils are fixed and the corneal, spinociliary, oculovestibular and oculocephalic reflexes are also absent. – The oculocephalic reflex is shown to be absent when passive movement of the head fails to elicit the normal response (present with intact brain stem function) of conjugate gaze to the opposite side.
- Oculovestibular reflexes are tested by irrigating the tympanic membrane on each with ice-cold water (ensuring first that the membrane is intact). A normal response is represented by mystagmus with the rapid component away from the irrigated side.

The tests are carried out by two independent clinicians and repeated after a period of, say, twenty-four hours. If there is any doubt regarding the influence of drugs or other metabolic factors, the tests should be deferred until such effects can be excluded.

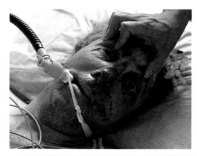

Fig. 110 Absent oculocephalic reflex.

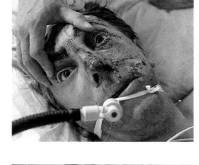

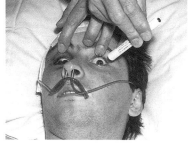

Fig. 111 Pupils tested for reaction to light.

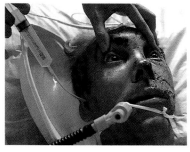

Fig. 112 Checking oculovestibular reflexes.

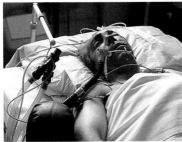

Fig. 113 After preoxygenation, artificial ventilation is temporarily suspended in the CO_2 stimulation test.

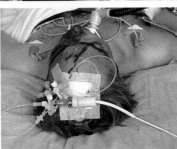

REHABILITATION

The long-term management of head injuries may require the expertise of physiotherapists, occupational and speech therapists and, possibly, specialized rehabilitation units. Patients with neurological deficits, including speech or limb disorders, may require retraining for new occupations and considerable support if mental problems and depression supervene.

A patient who has sustained a severe head injury may have his driver's licence revoked for one year, even if a full recovery is made within that period. Any patient with post-traumatic epilepsy has his licence revoked for a period of two years following the last fit; drivers of heavy goods vehicles have their licences revoked permanently. Patients should be advised that it is incumbent upon them to inform the Department Vehicle Licensing Centre (DVLC) of their injuries.

PREVENTION

The ideal solution to the problem of head injuries is to avoid them. It is important that the public be made aware of the safety measures available which help to avoid injuries to the head during sport or working activities. Stricter rules regarding drunken driving and the wearing of seatbelts have reduced the number of major injuries to the head in road traffic accidents, but there is still a great deal of progress to be made in industry and in sports, such as horse-riding, if even greater numbers of unnecessary catastrophies are to be prevented.

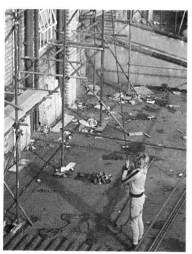

Fig. 114 At this site of recently completed building works, a man was having heavy objects thrown down to him from scaffolding about thirty feet above. Note his obvious lack of protective headgear.

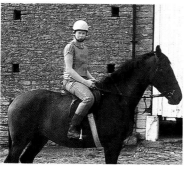

Fig. 115 A jockey's skull cap provides far more protection to the head when riding than the conventional riding hat. Many head injuries are caused by riders wearing a hat without a secure chin strap or not wearing one at all.

INDEX